STARS IN BALANCE

An Inspiring Guide That Lightens the Path of Those Embarking Into This New World of Girls Gymnasts

Jenny J. Jacques

The most important legacy you can leave is the positive impact you have on the lives of the people around you.

Thank you!

Dedicated with love to each of my grandchildren: Aleah, Liam, Mía, Amaya, Brielle, and to all the "Stars in Balance" who are the light of tomorrow.

Acknowledgement

AN INSPIRING AND PRACTICAL RESOURCE FOR YOUNG GYMNASTS, PARENTS, GRANDPARENTS, OR GUARDIANS THAT WILL ALLOW THEM TO UNDERSTAND, SUPPORT AND CELEBRATE THE CHALLENGES AND TRIUMPHS OF THEIR "STARS IN BALANCE" YOUNG PEOPLE.

Discover the beauty of gymnastics, the dedication it requires, and the spirit of your young athlete to progress in the world of gymnastics.

CONTENIDO

From:

....

To:

....

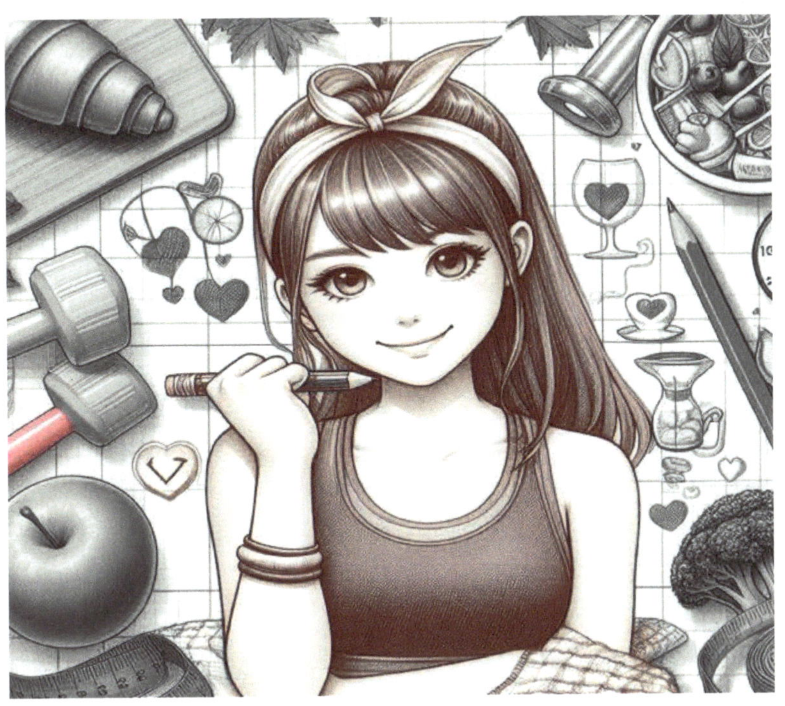

Affirmation:

"I am a Star in Balance shining in my own light."

Write your name here!

TO READ TOGETHER

Every girl or boy who has physical skills and who attends or wants to attend a gym should have a small guide that provides them with the basic knowledge to begin to expand their dreams beyond the gym they attend.

Although today there is a trend of talented and graceful female gymnasts, many attend gyms to develop their physical skills and in some cases to become professionals. Likewise, there are also few who acquire basic knowledge of this training, which in the very near future could become their lifestyle forever.

The truth is that the world of gymnasts is full of little stars with talent, dedication, and unforgettable stories.

There are many parents, grandparents and entire families who support their little girls to encourage their creativity, passion, and skill in the world of gymnastics through this sport.

I wrote this guide inspired by my little granddaughter Ali. Currently she is ten years old.

A few months after she was born, I realized that Ali had some ability to move, and when she just started crawling, she also started dancing. I remember my amazement at seeing her do her first dance steps that she learned from watching television.

It is true that children learn by imitation, but some are born with that gift, with that gift that is difficult not to appreciate with the naked eye.

In Ali's case, she became more agile and flexible over time. She never sat still, she was always tumbling, jumping, stretching, or dancing.

At seven years old, that whirlwind of energy of hers led her to want to practice different gymnastics and dance routines, but she found her love for Olympic gymnastics.

She is the oldest of four siblings. Her little brothers admire her and applaud all her practices and they also try hard to do all those pirouettes that Ali does so naturally.

She is very disciplined for her age, and she really wants to improve herself. She is a respectful, teachable, and talented girl, and in her practices she always concentrates on learning new techniques and giving the best of herself.

A few years ago, I was immersed in the world of Fitness. I used to exercise and spend hours in the gym training. When Ali was two years old, I remember taking her to the park many afternoons and exercising with her.

I learned to be aware of the harmony between the body, mind, and spirit, what can be achieved through exercise, and I managed to tune into these three dimensions where movement, breathing and heartbeat create a perfect rhythm.

When you exercise, the body releases all tension, the muscles stretch and strengthen, and the mind calms down, leaving everyday worries behind. It is as if the spirit rises and connects with something bigger, something more valuable than everything around you.

This knowledge and experience led me to admire all the people who dedicate themselves to different physical routines and sports. Each discipline is a testimony of determination, effort, dedication, and love for movement.

Each physical routine is a search for balance and connection with that something higher.

CHILDREN AND SPORTS

First seven years of a child are fundamental for their physical, mental, and emotional development. Because at this age they are learning to trust herself, explore the world and develop their own personality that is unique.

Between the ages of seven and fourteen they begin to look for a place in society and begin to face norms and rules imposed by parents, teachers and by their own environment.

Many children begin to question more than what they are taught, especially in these times where technology is available to everyone.

It is also a time when the child feels the need to find his or her own truth or sense of purpose. Here at this stage, it is essential to help them connect with the deepest values and foster an environment of love, trust, and openness so that they can explore the world in a healthy and authentic way.

Sport is a wonderful opportunity for play and exploration where children enjoy moving and participating when they are young, and where they also improve their skills, strategies and decision-making as they move into adolescence.

Children's mentality in sports is evolving from exploration and fun to competition, and it is important to encourage a positive attitude and a healthy approach towards sports at all ages.

My little Ali is interested in entering the Competition Group for next year, and I decided to write a guide for her.

I discovered that Ali needed to know a little more about everything she was living and experiencing at this stage of her life as a gymnast.

In February 2024, I traveled to Massachusetts and began doing extensive research to help Ali put together some points that were not very clear to her.

When Ali returned from school I surprised her with this gift, and to my surprise, I saw her face excited and happy when she read it.

It was Ali who asked me to publish this guide so that other girls like her could read it.

And I feel very grateful for that.

CREATING THE STORY OF YOUR LITTLE GYMNAST

There are wonderful inspiring stories of young champions and Olympic medal winners. All those young women full of talent and determination have left indelible marks in the hearts of many people. All of them were at some point girls with a big dream.

Those girls trained, got stronger and believed in themselves, showing the world what a girl with a big dream can achieve.

Parents: your support and love are essential. Help them to follow her dreams and fly high.

How can I support my little girl on her path?

You must be clear that self-confidence is the key in gymnastics.

- Believe in her abilities and in your little one's ability to overcome any obstacle. When you believe in her abilities, you are transmitting a message of confidence. You are telling her: "You can do it," so your girl will feel supported, valued, she will feel more confident and will be able to face challenges.

- You will be her motivating force and your little one will strive and persist even if things get difficult.

- Enjoy this shared time, enjoy their workouts. May everything, she do become a game combined with effort and grace.

- Create a positive environment where she can feel the support of her teammates, coaches, and family.

- Recognize and praise all her efforts, tell her not to worry if she can't do all the movements perfectly from the beginning, because each small advance will be an achievement to celebrate.

- Let her know and understand that there will be times when she will feel tired or frustrated, remind her why she started so she can keep going. Teach him that perseverance is the key to success.

- Help her dream big, work on her imagination, ask her to visualize herself doing her perfect routines in the scenario of her dreams. Tell her that all her dreams can come true.

- Motivate her, you can write notes with positive messages about exercise, and stick them on the mirror, on the back of her bed or in her playroom.

- Help her practice a daily routine at home on days he doesn't practice at the gym. Plan a small calendar for her activities.

- Stay active yourself, led by example.

- Promote healthy eating and explain how nutrition affects their energy levels and sports performance.

- Establish a regular sleep schedule, even on weekends.

- Restrict the use of electronic devices, TV, computer, laptops, at least one hour before bed. Blue light from screens can speed up your heart rate and make it difficult to sleep. Establishing good sleep habits is also part of living a healthy lifestyle.

- Ask her about his workouts. Pay attention when she shows you her new learnings. Get involved as a mother or father.

-Allow her to select her sports clothing within standards, she recognizes comfort in every movement.

- Read stories to her or let her watch stories about Olympic gymnasts.

Your patience and dedication as a father will be creating your own legacy.

Now make a ⊠ check mark on all the ones that apply.

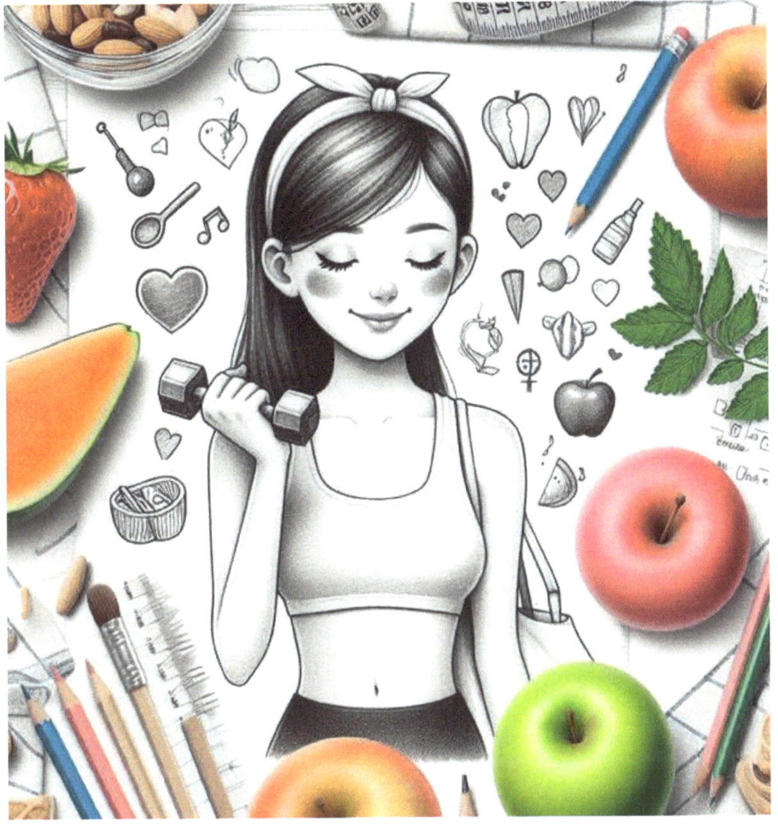

"Your children walk on the foundations of your love and sacrifice.

Write this story with love and courage."

A NATURAL GYMNAST

A natural gymnast is someone who displays natural gymnastic abilities. They have not had to go through a formal or structured training program.

We could say that they are those boys or girls who have the natural ability to perform gymnastic movements such as jumps, somersaults, acrobatics, or elasticity. They have ease, dexterity, and coordination to execute those movements with great grace.

While it is true, that all children can develop skills and enjoy gymnastics, there are others who can have a high level of skill without formal training and although this may seem like an initial advantage, they will also need constant training and practice to reach their maximum potential in this discipline.

It is important to find a local gym or club where the child can receive instruction from a professional. Having a good coach will help you improve your skills and develop your capabilities.

Constant practice can turn anyone into a master, expert or professional in their chosen field.

What may start as a game may be preparing her for the future, and if her also has the natural abilities from birth, her will need your support and the guidance of professional trainers.

FEATURES THAT STAND OUT

General knowledge

Physical strength: Gymnasts must constantly work on developing their muscular strength. This allows them to perform complex movements and maintain correct posture during routines.

Flexibility: Flexibility is essential to perform a variety of movements and postures in gymnastics.

Agility: Agility allows gymnasts to move quickly and easily, which is crucial for gymnastics routines.

Coordination: Coordination is necessary to perform complex movements and maintain balance.

Grace: Grace is important in gymnastics, especially rhythmic gymnastics, which integrates artistic elements such as dance or ballet steps into a body strength and flexibility exercise routine.

Balance and control: Gymnasts need good balance and control to perform precise movements and maintain balance during routines.

Endurance: Endurance is necessary to maintain a high level of performance during gym routines.

These characteristics are essential for any type of gymnastics, whether artistic, rhythmic, trampoline, acrobatic or aerobic.

TIPS FROM COACHES

1. Continue with training and discipline: Discipline and constant training are essential in gymnastics. You must continue to practice regularly and maintain your commitment to the sport.

2. Learn and practice the fundamentals: It is important that you learn and practice the basic movements of gymnastics, such as kites and bridges. These movements form the basis of more advanced skills.

3. Maintain a positive attitude: Attitude is key. You must maintain a positive attitude, even when things get difficult. Support and encouragement from those who love you can be very motivating.

4. Be careful with injuries: Gymnastics can be a high-risk sport, so it is important that you take precautions to avoid injuries. You must learn to perform the movements correctly and always warm up before training.

5. Improve your eating habits: Good nutrition is essential for young athletes. You should eat a balanced diet that includes enough protein, carbohydrates, and healthy fats. It is also important that you stay hydrated. Don't forget to drink water!

6. Work with a mentor or coach: They will give you guidance, teach you knew skills, and help you improve the techniques you've already learned.

7. READ THESE TIPS EVERY TIME YOU FEEL TIRED OR UNMOTIVED.

LEARNING A LITTLE HISTORY

The word "gymnastics" has its origins in Greek. It comes from the Greek word "gymnós," which is interpreted as "naked."

Gymnastics was born in ancient Greece. The Greeks were passionate about beauty and perfection and created this art that fused physical prowess with the very essence of humanity.

Their gyms were not places with modern machinery or televisions, but rather they were outdoor spaces, sunny places where young people gathered to train and connect with nature.

The most curious thing is that they did not wear clothes. They believed that nudity showed the natural beauty of their bodies.

In those gyms they learned all the physical skills, but they also learned history and culture.

Greeks held athletic competitions in honor of their gods. The Olympic Games were the most important and were in honor of Zeus, the most important god for the Greeks. But it wasn't just races and competitions, there was also music, poetry, and art.

Winning in those games was like receiving a hug from their gods and they were crowned with a crown of olive leaves.

Over time, gymnastics became popular, and the Romans also adopted it to improve the art of combat and the philosophy that united the mind and body.

Over the centuries, gymnastics evolved until it reached the elegant routines of artistic and rhythmic gymnastics that we see today.

Also today, gymnasts compete in the Olympic Games, a tradition that began more than 2,700 years ago, and in world championships, proving that the passion for beauty and perfection is still alive.

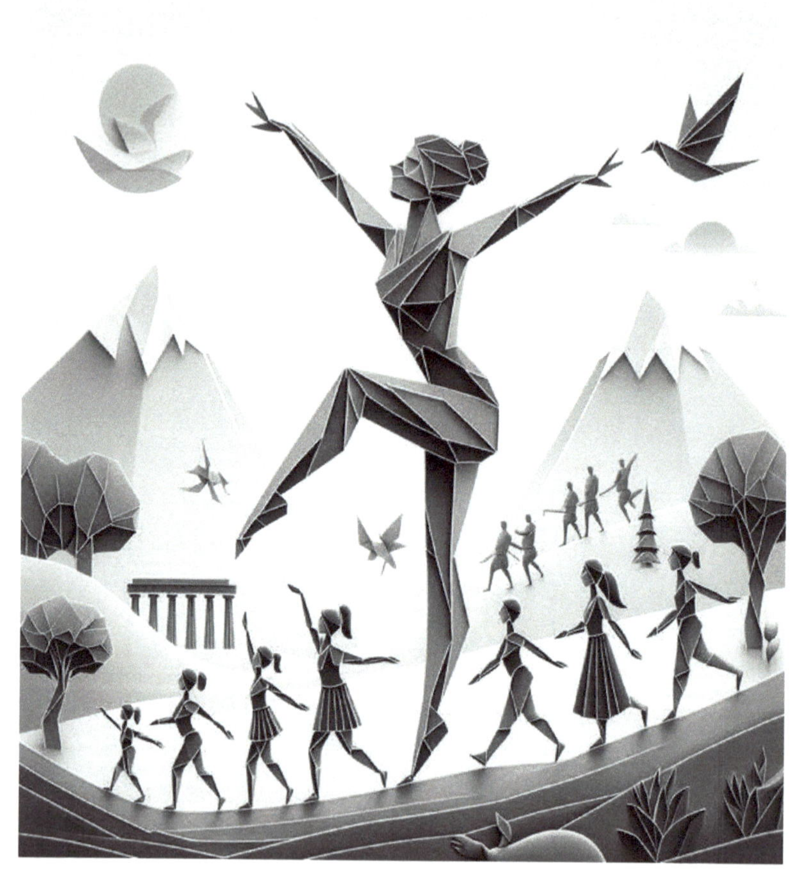

"*I wish that the grace, strength, and beauty of ancient athletes inspire you always.*"

THE IMPORTANCE OF CLOTHING "TODAY"

A gymnast's clothing plays an important role in the athlete's performance and comfort during exercise.

It is not a simple matter of fashion; it is much more important when it comes to selecting it.

Shall I explain to you why?

You are a gymnast jumping in the air and doing cartwheels and balance, that is very exciting! And your clothes should be like magic clothes.

It should be comfortable so that it fits well to your body and allows you to move without problems. Imagine if your t-shirt was too loose and got tangled while you jumped. That would be a real problem!

Also, the right clothing helps the muscles. Think of it as a gentle hug for your arms and legs that gives them strength and keeps them warm.

Now imagine that you are on a high bar or beam, if your clothes get caught it would be another problem.

That's why gymnasts wear tangle-free suits. Your gym suit should make you feel like a "Superhero," it should give you confidence and remind you that you are part of something big.

In short, your clothes should be comfortable, tight-fitting, and allow you freedom of movement.

CLOTHING DETAILS

Leotards or Bodysuits: Gymnasts usually wear leotards or bodysuits as their main clothing. Leotards can be short or long-sleeved and end in the groin area, very similar to the cut of a bikini.

Shorts: Although shorts are not allowed in competitions, they can be worn during training. They must be tight-fitting and have no elements that could cause injuries, such as pockets, threads, buttons, snaps, or zippers.

T-shirts: T-shirts are a comfortable option for male gymnasts in class. Like shorts, t-shirts are not allowed in competitions.

Long Gymnastics Pants: Gymnasts wear long gymnastics pants during competition and training.

Sports Bra: For women, it is advisable to wear a high-quality sports bra for good chest support.

Breathable Fabrics: Breathable fabrics allow good ventilation of the skin, preventing the accumulation of sweat and keeping the gymnast cool and dry during practice.

Remember, choosing the right clothing is essential to ensure the comfort, safety, and performance of the gymnast during gymnastics practice.

OLYMPIC GAMES: MOTIVATION AND ADVENTURE

Set your agenda, plan a special afternoon to watch the Olympic Games with your children, turn on the television and open the heart of your little gymnast.

Olympic Games are NOT JUST A COMPETITION, they are a symbol of unity, perseverance, and the search for the inner greatness of the human being.

Every movement, every jump, every tear, or celebration reminds us that we are part of something bigger in this world.

Behind every medal there is a dream achieved with a lot of sacrifice and dedication.

Struggles and victories of athletes are an inspiration to overcome our own limits.

Olympic Games remind us that, regardless of our differences, all human beings share the same dream of achieving greatness and leaving our mark on the history of life.

See athletes from all corners of the world, celebrating the diversity of cultures, languages and traditions with unique stories and brave hearts living their great purpose for humanity.

Make it a fun time while watching the game, you can do jumps or cartwheels in the room during commercials.

Talk about the athletes, explain that they have had to work very hard to get there. Talk to them about discipline, perseverance, and passion for what they do.

5 LAST OLYMPIC GAMES UNTIL 2024

1- London 2012 Olympic Games
Location: London, United Kingdom
Date: July 27 to August 12, 2012

2- Rio 2016 Olympic Games
Location: Rio de Janeiro, Brazil
Date: August 5 to 21, 2016

3- Pyeongchang 2018 Olympic Games
(Winter Games)
Location: Pyeongchang, South Korea.
Date: February 9 to 25, 2018

4- Tokyo 2020 Olympic Games (Held in
2021 due to the pandemic)
Location: Tokyo, Japan.
Date: July 23 to August 28, 2021

5- Paris 2024 Olympic Games
Location: Paris, France.
Date: July 26 to August 11, 2024

FOOD: THE MAGIC WAND OF A GYMNAST

Careful nutrition is essential for all children, but for a gymnast, it is even more important.

Your body is what has the energy to jump, spin and do stunts. It's like your body has magical powers. And you will need more energy to train and compete.

Only a good diet will provide you with that energy and carbohydrates will be like the gasoline your body needs.

Child gymnasts are also constantly growing and developing their bodies, and need nutrients to build strong bones, muscle, and tissue.

After an intense workout, the body needs to recover. Children should eat after each gymnastics section. To keep your body in good condition, you need to eat healthy foods.

Fruits, vegetables, and proteins are like magic potions for your body. Avoid junk foods, gymnasts need nutritious foods.

Parents and coaches should plan meals and snacks and should not skip important meals.

Drinking water is another magic potion, and you should not forget to drink it as it will keep you hydrated, fresh and full of energy.

Your body will need rest. Sleeping well will be like recharging all your magical powers.

So, eat well, drink water and rest so you can always be ready for action!

Note to parents: It is important to remember that each gymnast is unique and may have individual nutritional needs. You can develop a personalized meal plan with a sports dietician or health professional.

It is also necessary to have a regular physical examination with your primary doctor.

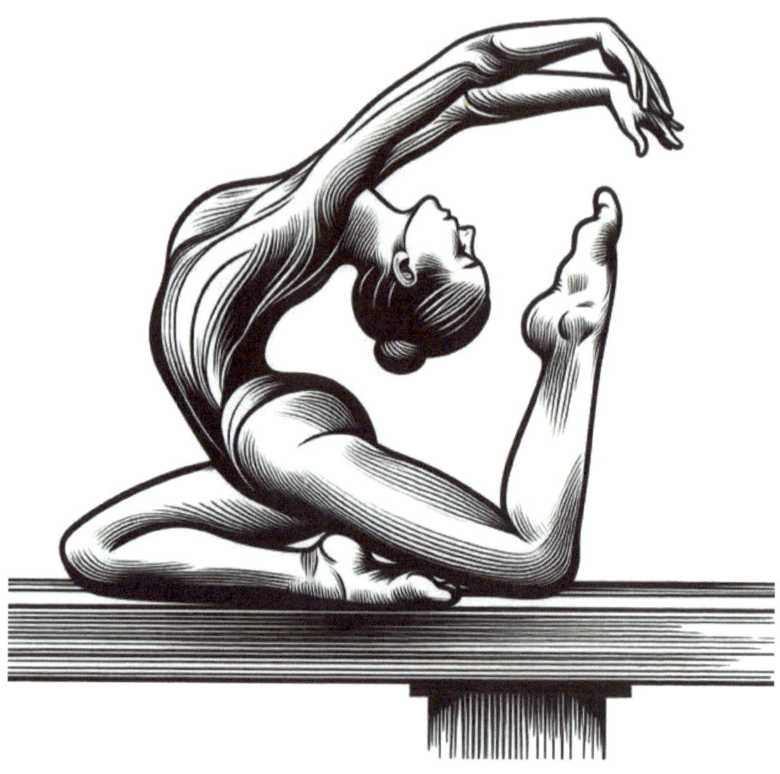

"Gymnastics is not about being better than everyone else. It's about being better than you used to be. Keep trying, keep trying, and keep believing in yourself."

FEEDING CHAMPIONS

Nutrition Behind an Athlete

Nutrition is essential for young gymnasts, providing the energy, nutrients, and minerals necessary for muscle growth, repair, and overall performance.

Without proper nutrition, gymnasts are more prone to injuries, may suffer frequent stress fractures, feel lethargic, have reduced performance, and develop amenorrhea or other hormonal imbalances.

Nutrition is beginning to play a more critical role in competitive and elite gymnastics as it directly affects the performance of the gymnast.

Olympic gymnasts typically train more than 30 hours a week, so a balanced diet can provide energy, support muscle development and repair, and improve endurance.

An ideal diet for a gymnast encompasses a balance of carbohydrates, proteins, iron, and fats:

Carbohydrates provide energy for muscle and brain function during high-intensity exercise and make up at least 50% of a gymnast's diet.

Proteins are essential for developing muscles and repairing tissues and the supply of iron is important and essential for muscle recovery and growth.

Fats are vital for brain health, nerve insulation and organ protection.

It is important to remember that each gymnast is unique and may have individual nutritional needs. Therefore, it is advisable to collaborate with a sports dietician or health professional to develop a personalized eating plan.

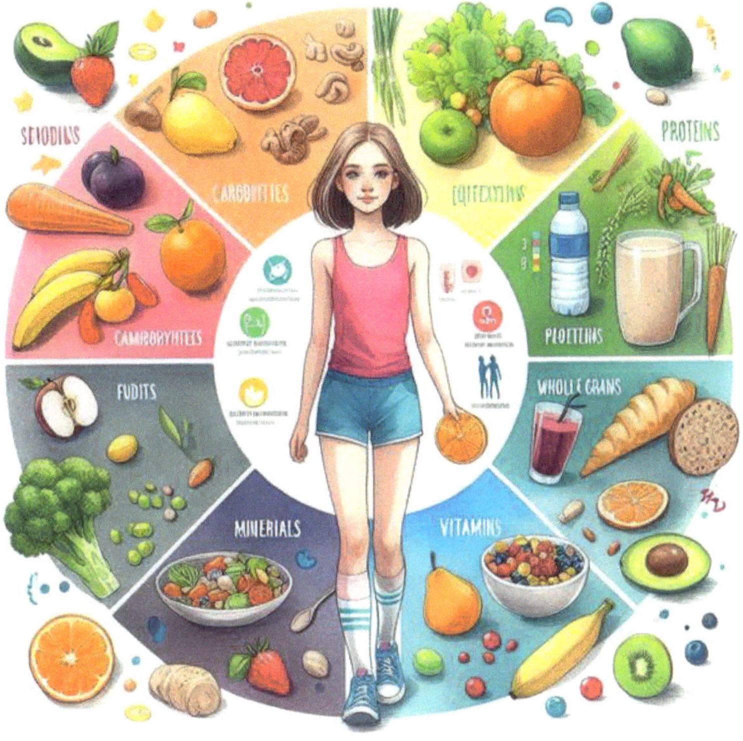

Avoid processed and high-sugar foods.

Foods that are good for gymnasts include a variety of essential nutrients to maintain their energy and support their performance.

Here are some examples:

Yogurt: It is an excellent source of calcium and vitamin D, essential for maintaining healthy bones. Greek yogurt is also a good source of protein.

Cheese: Like yogurt, cheese is an important source of calcium.

Cereals: Whole grains are an excellent source of carbohydrates, which provide energy for training and competition.

Nuts: They are a good source of healthy fats and proteins.

Colorful Vegetables: They provide a wide range of vitamins and minerals.

Fibrous Fruits: Fruits are an excellent source of carbohydrates and dietary fiber.

High-quality Protein: Lean meats, chicken, fish, and eggs are excellent sources of protein.

Salmon: It is an excellent source of protein and omega-3 fatty acids.

Starches: Foods like potatoes and rice are a good source of carbohydrates.

Fun Foods: Including foods you enjoy can help maintain a healthy relationship with food.

According to sports dietician Christina Anderson, a specialist in gymnast nutrition, she says on her blog that a gymnast who trains fifteen to thirty hours a week will need two to three extra snacks to improve energy and training levels. The snack should be a mini meal, a combination of carbohydrates that provide energy and stabilize blood glucose.

She also says that snacks cannot replace three meals a day.

You can find more information on her personal blog: I recommend it https://christinaandersonrdn.com

5 HEALTHY SNACK IDEAS

1. Banana and Peanut Butter Toast: It is an excellent option for a snack full of proteins and carbohydrates.
2. Greek Yogurt with Fruits and Nuts: Greek yogurt is rich in protein and can be combined with fresh fruits and nuts to add fiber and healthy fats.
3. Hummus with Vegetable Sticks: Hummus is a source of protein and fiber, and can be served with carrots, cucumbers, or peppers.
4. FruitS and Protein Shake: A shake of protein powder and your favorite fruits can be an excellent option for after training.
5. Homemade Granola Bars: You can make your own granola bars with oats, nuts, seeds, and honey. They are an excellent source of energy and are easy to take to the gym.
6. Write your favorite snack here!

....

....

....

....

Again, I remind you that each gymnast is unique and may have unique nutritional needs. That is why it is advisable to collaborate with a sports dietitian or health professional to develop a personalized eating plan.

A LITTLE STORY TO READ BEFORE GOING TO SLEEP

"THE GIFT OF ...." (write your name)

There once was a girl named ....

From the moment she was born, everyone noticed something special about her.

She had endless energy and amazing flexibility not often seen in a baby. Her parents and her grandmother soon realized that she had a special gift for gymnastics.

As she grew, her love for gymnastics grew as well.

She spent hours practicing in the yard or in her playroom, perfecting her skills and learning new routines.

 She demonstrated dedication and discipline that went beyond her younger years.

When she turned ...... years old, she joined a local gymnastics team. Despite being the youngest, she quickly stood out for her talent and ability. Her coach, impressed by her dedication and natural ability, encouraged her to compete in national competitions.

She worked tirelessly, training every day after school and on weekends. Despite her challenges and difficulties, she never gave up. She knew she had a special gift and was determined to do everything she could to reach her full potential.

Finally, she arrived on the day of the national competition. She was nervous but excited.

 When it was her turn, she stood in the center of the stage, took a deep breath, and began her routine. With every jump and spin, the crowd was amazed. Her performance was impeccable, and at the end of her routine, the room erupted in applause.

...Won the competition that day, but for her, the real prize was the trip. Through her dedication and love for gymnastics, she had proven that, with hard work and determination, anything is possible.

Since then, she has continued to compete, but most importantly she continues to love gymnastics.

Good rest!

"I AM WHO I AM TODAY BECAUSE OF MANY THINGS I LEARNED IN GYMNASTICS."

Katelyn Ohashi

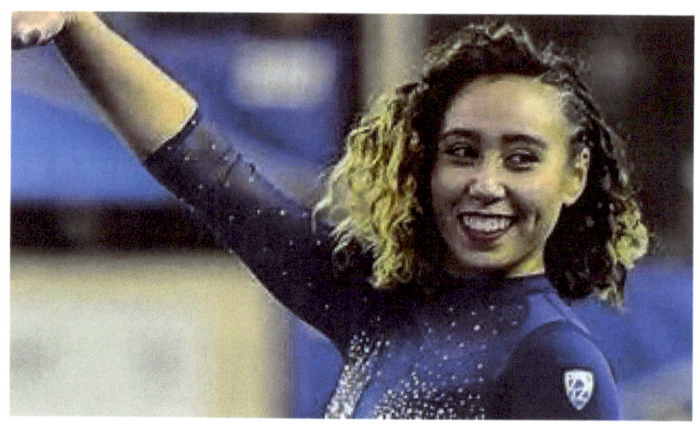

Katelyn Michelle Ohashi is a former American artistic gymnast who competed for the University of California, Los Angeles (UCLA). She was born on April 12, 1997, in Seattle, Washington1. She is a six-time All-American and was a four-time USA Gymnastics junior national team member, 2011 junior national champion, and 2013 America's Cup winner.

Ohashi is known for incorporating elements of folk dance into her floor routines1. In January 2019, she went viral on various social media sites for her perfect 10 score at the 2019 College Challenge, the fourth perfect ten floor routine of her career[1].

After retiring from gymnastics in 2019, Ohashi now spends her time as a social media star, participating in brand partnerships, writing, photography, and participating in the charity Project Heal. Despite no longer competing, she is still involved with her sport in various ways[2].

1. Wikipedia.org
2. Sportskeeda.com
3. Katelyn Ohashi – The official website for gymnast Katelyn Ohashi (katelyn-ohashi.com)

"GYMNASTICS TAUGHT ME EVERYTHING: LIFE LESSONS, RESPONSIBILITY, DISCIPLINE AND RESPECT."

Shawn Johnson

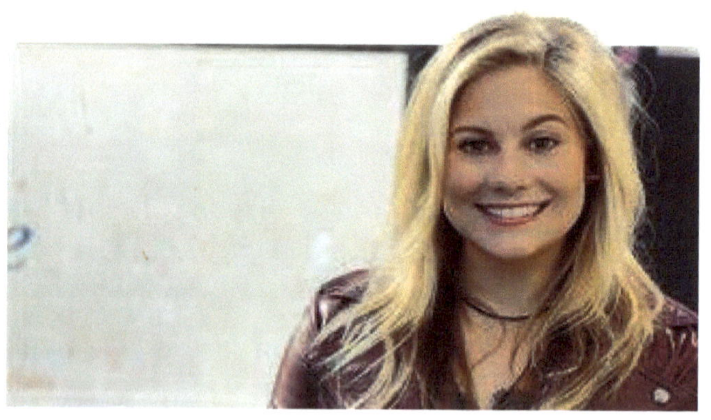

Shawn Johnson East, born Shawn Machel Johnson, is a former American artistic gymnast. She was born on January 19, 1992, in Des Moines, Iowa. She is the gold medalist on the balance beam at the 2008 Olympics and silver medalist in the team, individual competition, and floor routine[1]. Johnson is also the 2007 Individual World Champion and a five-time Pan American Games gold medalist, winning the team titles in 2007 and 2011[1].

In addition to her gymnastics career, Johnson has had success in other areas. In May 2009, she won the eighth season of "Dancing with the Stars," and in November 2012, she took second place in the all-star edition1. After retiring from gymnastics in 2012, Johnson became a certified Nike trainer. She has also written several books, including a New York Times Best Seller.

In her personal life, Johnson has been married to Andrew East since 2016. Together, they have built a significant presence on social media and continue to share their life and experiences with their followers[2].

1- Wikipedia.org
2- Shawnjohnson.com
3- Gymnastics | Shawn Johnson East | Traces of Gold

"YOU JUST HAVE TO BE YOURSELF AND HAVE FULL CONFIDENCE AND COURAGE."

Gabby Douglas

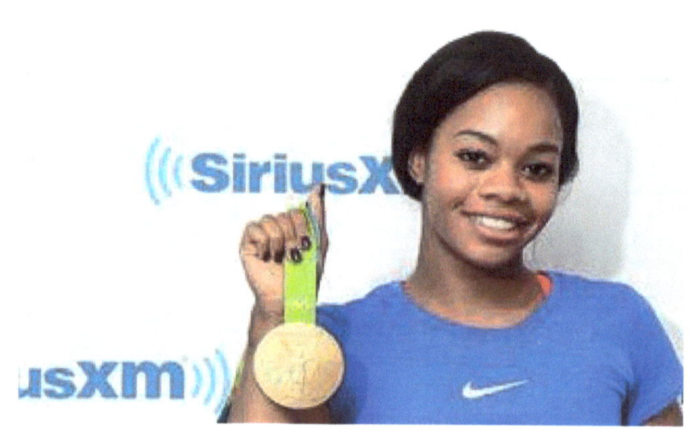

Gabrielle Christina Victoria Douglas, known as Gabby Douglas, is a former American artistic gymnast1. She was born on December 31, 1995, in Newport News, Virginia[1]. She is the 2012 Olympic champion in the individual competition and the 2015 world silver medalist in the same category[1]. She was a member of the gold-winning teams at the 2012 and 2016 Summer Olympics, nicknamed "Fierce Five" and "Final Five" by the media, respectively[1]. She was also a member of the United States gold-winning teams at the 2011 and 2015[1] World Championships.

Douglas is the first African American to become the individual Olympic champion in the history of the Olympic Games[1]. She is also the first American gymnast to win gold in both the individual and team competitions at the same Olympic Games1. Additionally, she was the champion of the 2016 AT&T America's Cup1.

Following her career in gymnastics, Douglas has found success in other areas. Her life and accomplishments were adapted into the 2014 Lifetime biopic, "The Gabby Douglas Story." She has also written a book about her life and what it takes to be an Olympic gold medalist through determination and perseverance1.

Recently, after almost eight years away from the sport that crowned her Olympic champion, Gabby Douglas has returned to gymnastics with her sights set on the Paris 2024 Olympic Games. If she manages to qualify, she will be the oldest American woman to compete in the gymnastics category since the 1950s[2].

1- Wikipedia.org
2- Nbcnews.com
3- Gabby Douglas: Olympic Gymnast (gabrielledouglas.com)

"I LEARNED THAT YOU DON'T HAVE TO WIN FIRST PLACE TO WIN."

Kim Zmeskal

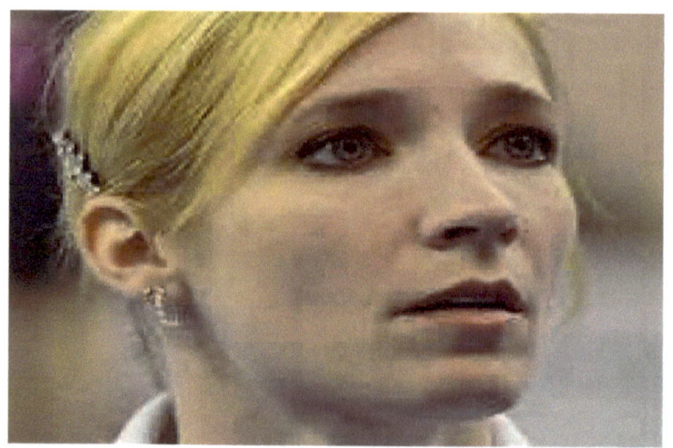

Kimberly Lynn Zmeskal Burdette, known as Kim Zmeskal, is a former American artistic gymnast1. She was born on February 6, 1976, in Houston, Texas[1]. She is the 1991 world champion in the individual[1] competition. She was a member of the US team that won the silver medal at the 1991 World Championships, the first team medal won by US women at a world championships[1]. She is also the 1992 world champion on the balance beam and floor exercise1. She was a member of the USA team that won the bronze medal at the 1992 Summer Olympics in Barcelona, Spain[1].

Zmeskal is known for her explosive power and tumbling in the vault and on the floor[1]. She is considered one of the greatest female gymnasts of all time and possibly the best in the world in the early 1990s. Her victory in the individual competition also marked the beginning of a dynasty of American dominance in women's gymnastics.

After retiring from gymnastics, Zmeskal became a gymnastics coach1. She currently owns Texas Dreams Gymnastics in Coppell, Texas, and hosts Kim Zmeskal's Texas Prime1 meet annually.

1- Wikipedia.com
2- Kim ZMESKAL (olympics.com)

LESSONS FOR LIFE AND PERSONAL GROWTH.

1. You should know that sometimes there will be triumphs and sometimes there will be defeats, and it is better that you learn it now. A defeat is not a failure, it is something temporary. If you don't give up and continue, what follows is success. Every successful person has had to face defeat at some point.
2. Set personal objectives and goals and move towards them.
3. Don't meddle in other people's lives and don't compare yourself to others. You are unique and special. A successful person doesn't have time for that. Focus.
4. Acquire adequate education and teaching. If you see that something is not correct, talk to your parents, teachers, or coaches.
5. Discipline in nutrition is as important as the opportunities that will be presented to you throughout life.
6. Having ambition is not bad, wanting to win and improve is good.
7. Having a positive mental attitude (positive thoughts) improves health.

8. Choose your friends well. Surround yourself with friends who share your aspirations and are happy about your achievements.
9. Always remember: every effort has a reward. Always go the extra mile.
10. Learn to make good decisions and ignore criticism.
11. Live in harmony and cooperate with others.
12. Expand your imagination and dream big, always imagine the best, and the best will come.
13. Be a loyal and sincere friend, even if others are not.
14. And most importantly, learn to forgive, although it may seem difficult, never try to take revenge on anyone. In life everyone gets what they give.

I wish you a life full of laughter, joy, and unforgettable moments. May opportunities abound in your life, to grow, learn and love.

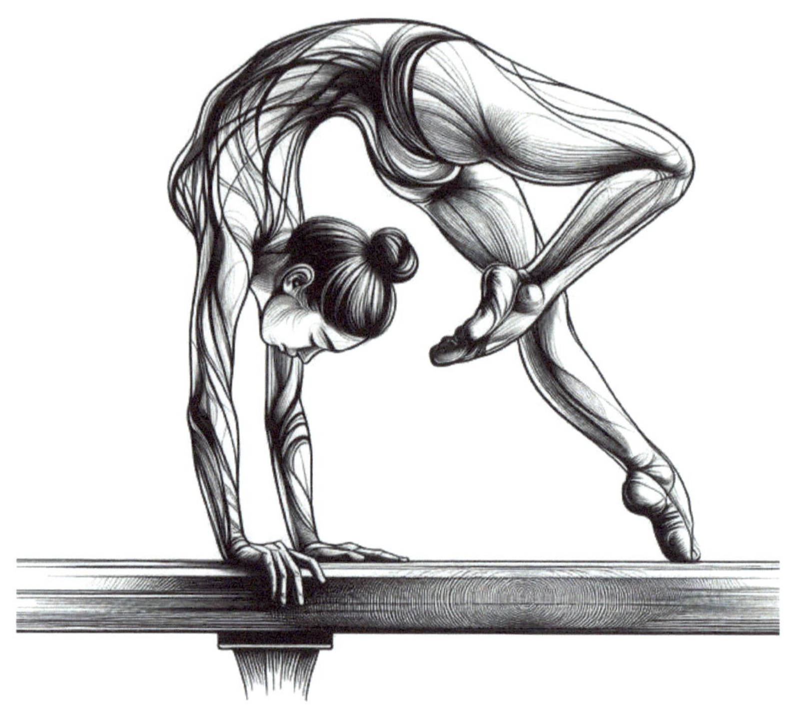

"ALI'S GIFT"

"Perfection is not about controlling every movement, but about having the courage to let go and trust yourself." Remember, gymnastics is not just a sport. It is a journey of self-discovery and confidence in your gifts.

If you liked it and want to share your personal story or tell me how this guide helped you, write me at: jen4ever1111@gmail.com

I'll be happy to read you. Thank you!

About the Author

Jenny J. Jacques was born in Uruguay, where she married and had three children. At the age of thirty-one, she immigrated to the United States to provide a better life for her family.

After going through difficult times after her divorce, Jenny focused all her energy on her personal transformation.

She trained for several years in the gym, achieving personal goals of physical transformation and finding the balance that would change the course of her life.

Despite her difficulties, Jenny continued to move forward, becoming the best version of herself to be able to help other people, especially in times of pandemic, where she provided emotional support to a large group of women.

She has read over 200 books and listened to hundreds of audiobooks on Personal Growth and Spirituality over the years.

She has also trained with great mentors in these areas.

She considers herself a "lightworker" after a wonderful awakening of consciousness that connected her with her divine purpose in 2018.

She loves sports and admires those who dedicate their lives to any sporting discipline.

Her family plays an important role in her life, and she is very proud of her beautiful grandchildren.

This book, "Stars in Balance" is inspired by her eldest granddaughter, whom Jenny deeply admires for her athletic gifts.

Currently, Jenny works as a Life Coach, working alongside her husband, helping people reach their full potential so they can live full and satisfying lives.

Through her experience in *personal growth, spiritual growth, and professional growth,* she helps people manage stress, make decisions, find their life purpose, and improve their interpersonal relationships.

She understands the personal needs of this time and her coaching sessions are very effective.